What you really need to know about

LIVING WITH
DIABETES

Dr Robert Buckman

with Chris McLaughlin

Introduced by John Cleese

A QUANTUM BOOK

This edition published by Silverdale Books,
an imprint of Bookmart Ltd,
Blaby Road, Wigston, Leicester, LE18 4SE

This book is produced by
Quantum Publishing Ltd.
6 Blundell Street
London N7 9BH

ISBN 1-84573-131-X

QUM997

Printed in Singapore by
Star Standard Industries Pte Ltd

The consultant for this book was Simon O'Neill, Head of Care
at the
British Diabetic Association

Contents

Foreword

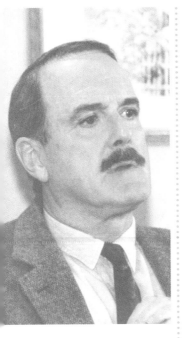

Most of you know me best as someone who makes people laugh.

But for 30 years I've also been involved with communicating information. And one particular area in which communication often breaks down is the doctor/patient relationship. We have all come across doctors who baffle instead of clarify, use complex medical terms when a simple explanation would do, and dismiss us with a "come back in a month if you still feel unwell". Fortunately, I met Dr Robert Buckman.

Rob is one of North America's leading experts on cancer, but far more importantly he is a doctor who believes that hiding behind medical jargon is unhelpful and unprofessional. He wants his patients to understand what is wrong with them, and spends many hours with them—and their families and close friends—making sure they understand everything. Together we created a series of videos, with the jargon-free title *Videos for Patients*. Their success has prompted us to write books that explore medical conditions in the same clear, simple terms.

This book is one of a series that will tell you all you need to know about your condition. It assumes nothing. If you have a helpful, honest, communicative doctor, you will find here the extra information that he or she may not have time to tell you. If you are less fortunate, this book will help to give you a clearer picture of your situation.

More importantly—and this was a major factor in the success of the videos—you can access the information here again and again. Turn back, read over, until you really know what your doctor's diagnosis means. In addition, because in the middle of a consultation, you may not think of everything you would like to ask your doctor, you can also use the book to help you formulate the questions you would like to discuss with him or her.

John Cleese

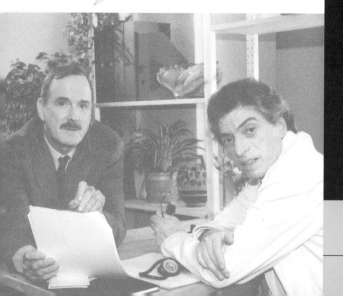

Introduction

DID YOU KNOW?

Diabetes used to be known as "sugar diabetes" possibly because of the sweet smell on the breath of the sufferer.

Sugar is in fact sucrose (refined from cane or beet) while the one in the blood is glucose made by the body from food.

All brain and red blood cells must have a constant supply of glucose to survive.

Finding out that you have diabetes can come as a shock, and it usually takes a while to absorb the news and all the implications. At the moment, there is no cure, which means facing up to the prospect of living with the condition and possibly needing treatment for the rest of your life. It's only natural to worry about what this will mean, how you will be able to cope and what effect it will have on your life and those of your family and friends.

Information and support

The first thing to remember is that you will not be left to cope on your own. The doctor who is caring for you— whether it's your GP or a hospital consultant and his or her team—will explain the condition in detail and discuss the most appropriate form of treatment.

You will also be able to call upon the expertise of a range of other health professionals, including diabetes specialist nurses, dietitians and podiatrists as and when you need them. You will be encouraged to learn as much as you can about your condition and what you can do to help yourself stay in the best possible health.

Feeling better

A few people who develop diabetes later in life will not have noticed any symptoms prior to diagnosis, but most people find they start to feel much better once treatment has brought their condition under control. You may well find that you have much more energy and start to feel really on top again in a way that you haven't done for a long time. If you are able to follow the lifestyle advice you are given, including taking exercise, eating well and, if necessary, losing weight and giving up smoking, you will find that not only is it easier to manage your diabetes, but you will feel generally fitter and healthier than you did before. Don't expect too much of yourself too quickly—it will take a while to adjust and to introduce the necessary changes. Take it one step at a time.

A normal life

You will be given advice about the right kind of diet—which is likely to be far more enjoyable than you might have expected—and many people will also start on tablets or insulin treatment. Even if you have to inject yourself with insulin, you will find that it is really quite simple and painless once you have got the hang of it. Within a relatively short time, most people can adapt to living with diabetes and find that their condition places few if any restrictions on their lifestyle.

The secret of controlling the condition is to work in partnership with your medical advisers. The more you understand about diabetes and its management, the better! The members of your diabetes care team understand that you will need to take time to learn about your condition and won't mind at all if you have to have the same question answered several times. Never hesitate to consult them when you need support.

THE BRITISH DIABETIC ASSOCIATION

Many people find the information and other services provided for members by the British Diabetic Association invaluable. You can also make contact with your local BDA group where you will meet other people who are living with diabetes. You'll find more details on page 78.

Chapter

SYMPTOMS & CAUSES

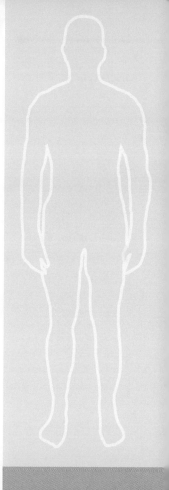

What is diabetes?

FACTS

✓ People with diabetes have too much glucose in their bloodstream.

✗ The disease is brought on because not enough insulin is produced to turn the glucose into energy.

The full name of the condition, *diabetes mellitus*, comes from Greek words meaning "a fountain of sugar". This is because physicians in the ancient world noticed that people with diabetes produced lots of sweet urine, although they did not know why.

We now understand how sugar levels are regulated by the body. Starchy (carbohydrate) foods in the diet are broken down by the digestive system into glucose and released into the bloodstream. When glucose levels rise, the pancreas releases a hormone called insulin which enables the body cells to absorb glucose to use as a source of energy. Any which is not needed immediately is stored in the liver or as fat and can be released when required—to fuel muscles during exercise, for example, or during long periods without food.

THE INSULIN/GLUCOSE CYCLE

As the digestive system releases glucose into the bloodstream, the healthy pancreas secretes just the right amount of insulin needed to handle it. The blood glucose level then falls, and insulin release is switched off until you eat again. The system is perfectly balanced to keep blood glucose levels within a narrow range at all times.

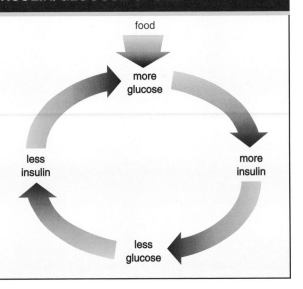

food

more glucose

more insulin

less glucose

less insulin

CHILDREN AND DIABETES

Occasionally very young children can develop insulin-dependent diabetes, even in the first few weeks of life. However, with the right help and support, parents can learn to manage the illness successfully.

The system is so well-balanced by the body that the level of glucose in the blood stays fairly constant, unless something goes wrong. People with diabetes have too much glucose in their bloodstream because the normal control mechanism regulating the balance of insulin and glucose is not working as it should. As a result the body is unable to process all the circulating glucose in the blood in the normal way, leading to a rise in the blood sugar levels. Some of the excess sugar is removed by the kidneys and excreted in the urine.

Until the early part of the 20th century, when insulin and its effect on the body were first identified, there was no treatment for the disease and people with the condition eventually died. Now it is possible to take steps to regulate glucose levels artificially, through drugs or by controlling the diet.

Because in diabetes normal feedback mechanisms no longer work properly, you can't rely on nature to supply the right amount of insulin in response to blood glucose levels. You have to try to create this balance yourself through the food you eat—regular meals and snacks—and exercise together with medication in many cases. By manipulating these elements it is possible to gain good control over your diabetes.

◆ Carbohydrate foods are turned into glucose which is needed for immediate energy or stored.

◆ In a healthy body the right amount of insulin is produced to keep glucose levels in the blood normal.

◆ People with diabetes need help so that their blood glucose levels stay within a healthy range.

What is diabetes?

What goes wrong?

There are two distinct forms of diabetes mellitus. In young people it is the result of a failure of the insulin supply. However, the most common type develops in middle or later life and is usually the result of a change in the body's ability to respond to insulin which is called "insulin resistance". In these people insulin production may also be less effective than normal.

Type 1 diabetes

The first way in which the process of glucose and insulin control can be disrupted by diabetes is when the cells in the pancreas which secrete insulin—the beta cells in the Islets of Langerhans—stop working. This failure of the person's own supply means they have to replace it with insulin given by injection and they are therefore said to have type 1 (insulin-dependent) diabetes.

Although this is probably the best-known form of the condition, it is actually not the most common. It usually comes on before the age of 40, and often during childhood or adolescence.

Type 2 diabetes

Type 2 diabetes is also known as late-onset diabetes or non-insulin-dependent diabetes, though in fact some people who have it are treated with insulin.

This more common form of diabetes results from something going wrong with the way the person's body handles insulin. It is believed that the person becomes resistant to insulin so that it is less effective at its task of enabling the body to absorb glucose from the bloodstream. Such people may also be producing reduced amounts of insulin, but their supply does not fail completely as in type 1.

Type 2 diabetes normally develops later in life and is particularly common in people who are overweight. Unlike insulin-dependent diabetes, it develops gradually and you may not notice anything for some time unless you are alert for possible symptoms.

Initially you will probably try dietary changes alone, but if these are not sufficient, your doctor will probably suggest tablet treatment. If none of the oral medications work, then insulin will be considered.

HOW INSULIN IS PRODUCED

The pancreas is a long, thin gland which sits behind the stomach just above the liver. One area of cells within the pancreas—called the Islets of Langerhans—is responsible for producing insulin and also another hormone which triggers the release of a form of glucose, called glycogen, when blood glucose levels drop too low.

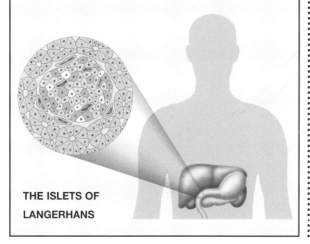

THE ISLETS OF LANGERHANS

◆ You can have type 2 diabetes without being aware of it.

◆ Only a minority of people need to have insulin injections to control their blood glucose levels.

◆ Overweight people are more likely to develop diabetes later in life.

What goes wrong?

How is your body affected?

SELF HELP

Keep all your check-ups or appointments at your GP's surgery or hospital clinic so that any early signs of complications are spotted.

The British Diabetic Association can offer support and advice and put you in touch with other people with the condition.

Higher than normal levels of glucose in the blood for more than very brief periods can affect many parts of the body adversely. Some of these problems may take years to develop, but making sure that your blood glucose stays within the normal limits as far as humanly possible makes them far less likely to occur at all. This is one of the main reasons why maintaining good control is vital.

THE EFFECTS OF DIABETES

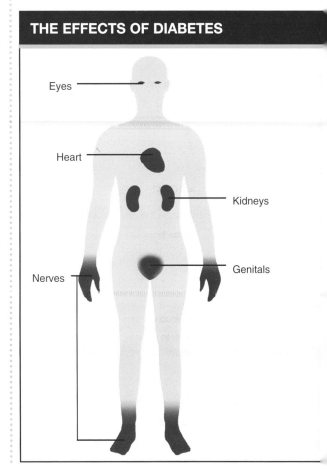

Eyes

Heart

Kidneys

Genitals

Nerves

Nerves and blood vessels

Many of the long-term complications relate to the damage to nerve and/or blood vessels caused by raised —and uncontrolled—levels of blood glucose. Nerve damage is called neuropathy by the medical profession. It can affect nerves in any part of the body, but it is mostly likely to cause problems with your feet.

EYES

Diabetic retinopathy is the result of changes in the blood vessels of the eye which can affect sight.

HEART

People with diabetes are vulnerable to circulatory problems, which can narrow the coronary arteries, causing angina and increasing the risk of a heart attack.

KIDNEYS

People with high blood glucose levels are prone to cystitis, bladder and kidney infections, and diabetes can result in damage to small blood vessels.

NERVES

Damage to nerves and small blood vessels can cause numbness and lack of sensitivity to pain. As a result you may be unaware of minor injuries, which can then become infected.

GENITALS

Uncontrolled diabetes can cause itching in the genital area. In men damage to the blood vessels supplying the penis can lead to impotence.

YOU REALLY NEED TO KNOW

◆ Blood glucose levels that are uncontrolled are the main reason for long-term complications.

◆ Damage to the nerves and blood vessels occurs slowly but can ultimately cause very serious problems.

◆ Some over-the-counter remedies can affect blood glucose levels, so always check with the pharmacist.

The problem areas

✓ Regular eye checks which look at the backs of the eyes are essential. Eye problems can be treated effectively if diagnosed early.

✓ If you wear glasses, regular sight tests will pick up any deterioration. But don't change your prescription within 3 months of diagnosis.

✗ Avoid exposing your feet to extremes of temperature and take prompt action for any skin injury.

Some people may be more likely to experience complications because of their genetic make-up, but no one knows this for sure. It means that everyone with diabetes needs to be aware of the potential risks.

Heart disease

The fact that most people who develop non-insulin-dependent diabetes do so in their fifties or sixties means they may be at increased risk of circulatory problems, especially coronary heart disease. By this time of life, many people already have some degree of hardening of the arteries, which happens to all of us to some extent as we get older, and they may have also accumulated fatty deposits on the inside of their arteries. Raised blood glucose can exacerbate both these conditions, probably because it alters the balance of certain fats, such as cholesterol, in the blood.

Eyes

If your blood glucose was high for some time before your diabetes was diagnosed, you may notice that your distance vision improves once treatment has brought down your blood glucose levels. This is because raised glucose changes the shape of the lens and interferes with its ability to focus properly. People who have had diabetes for many years may suffer damage to the blood vessels at the back of the eyes, especially if the condition has not been well-controlled.

Impotence

Men who have had poorly-controlled diabetes for some years may become impotent as a result of damage to the nerves and blood supply to the penis.

Kidneys

One of the reasons you are asked for a urine sample at your check-ups is so that it can be tested for traces of protein which might indicate the beginnings of kidney problems. The presence of protein can be caused by damage to the small blood vessels or by an infection.

Legs and feet

Diabetes has the potential to accelerate hardening of the arteries which can result in a poor blood supply to the feet and fingers. This increases your susceptibility to such problems as infections and neuropathy, and may make you more sensitive to extremes of heat and cold.

DIABETES AND SIGHT

In people with type 2 diabetes the walls of the tiny capillaries at the back of the eye develop aneurisms (swellings) which burst, causing bleeding into the retina. Damage can be halted, not reversed, by laser treatment.

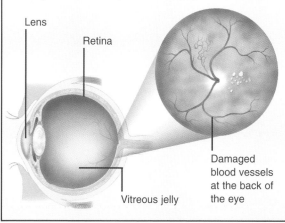

Lens

Retina

Damaged blood vessels at the back of the eye

Vitreous jelly

The problem areas

17

What causes diabetes?

There are over 2 million people with diabetes in the UK, but almost half are undiagnosed. No one actually knows why some people develop diabetes and others don't but there are likely to be several factors involved.

The causes of type 1 diabetes are thought to be different from those of type 2. In fact, some researchers also believe there may be subtle distinctions to be made between people who have type 2 diabetes in that their condition is brought about in slightly different ways.

Inherited factors

Although the genes you inherit from both your parents may play a part in determining whether you get diabetes, it isn't a straightforward inherited disease, in the way that haemophilia or cystic fibrosis are. The genetic link is also thought to be stronger in type 2 diabetes.

Bear in mind that having a close relative with diabetes does not mean you are bound to get it. In fact many people with the condition know of no close family members who are similarly affected. Nevertheless, diabetes is so common in this country that it wouldn't be altogether surprising if one of your relatives has it as well as you. It's probable that what you inherit is a susceptibility to the condition, and whether you ever get it will depend on other factors. In young people, the

WHAT ABOUT TWINS?

If you have an identical twin with type 2 diabetes, you are very likely to get it too. However, if he or she has type 1 diabetes, the odds are only 50/50.

1

FACTS AND FIGURES

◆ There are around 1.4 million people with diabetes in the UK, and an estimated million more who have the non-insulin-dependent type (type 2) but don't know it.

◆ Type 2 diabetes is more common than type 1, making up over 80 percent of the total of people with diabetes.

trigger may well be a virus (mumps and the Coxsackie group are among the suspects) but there is, as yet, insufficient evidence to be certain.

Non-inherited factors

In older people, weight and diet may be a significant factor since most people who develop type 2 diabetes are overweight.

There are geographical factors, with some areas having a higher incidence of diabetes than others. This may be partly due to diet and/or environmental factors.

Some illnesses may make you more likely to develop diabetes, including those which alter the balance of other hormones in your body. Culprits can include thyroid disease and Cushing's syndrome, inflammation of the pancreas and cystic fibrosis.

Another condition, diabetes insipidus, is a rare disorder of the pituitary gland in the brain. While it may also cause some similar symptoms, it is completely unrelated to the more common diabetes mellitus.

Drinking excessive amounts of alcohol can damage the pancreas and so cause diabetes.

YOU REALLY NEED TO KNOW

◆ Having a close relative with diabetes does not mean you are bound to get it too, but it may increase the odds, especially of type 2.

◆ A virus infection may bring on type 1 in people with a genetic tendency to develop it.

◆ Pancreas damage which occurs as a result of drinking excessive alcohol can bring on diabetes.

What causes diabetes?

Diabetes and pregnancy

✓ A regular exercise routine will encourage your system to use blood glucose efficiently. Ask your midwife if you are not sure what kind is best.

✗ Don't eat for two. It isn't necessary and you will gain weight that may increase the risk of gestational diabetes.

✗ Do not be tempted to skip an antenatal check, especially in the later part of your pregnancy.

A few women (about 3 percent) develop what is called gestational diabetes during pregnancy. The exact cause is unknown, but it is thought that it may be related to the hormones produced during pregnancy. After about the 24th week, the hormones secreted by the placenta (which links the blood supply of the mother to the growing baby) may make the pregnant woman's own insulin supply less effective so that she develops raised levels of glucose in her blood. The excess glucose overflows into her urine and will be detected in the routine tests done at the antenatal clinic.

Anyone who is thought to be particularly at risk of developing gestational diabetes (for example, someone who had the problem during a previous pregnancy) will probably be tested earlier in the pregnancy.

The mother's blood glucose returns to normal once the baby and the placenta have been delivered, but the woman is likely to have a similar problem if she becomes pregnant again. About half of those women who have gestational diabetes go on to develop type 2 diabetes later in life; their doctors should make periodic checks for diabetes.

Because a woman does not develop gestational diabetes in one pregnancy does not mean that she will not do so in subsequent pregnancies. In fact, as you get older your chances of developing the problem increase.

The effects on mother and baby

The baby receives its nourishment from the mother's blood supply via the placenta. If there is too much glucose in her bloodstream, the baby's body will produce extra insulin in response. This encourages fat storage and causes him or her to grow too big (a

CAN DIABETES EVER BE PREVENTED?

Medical science has no means as yet of preventing the disease developing in those most likely to get it. Research is underway to develop blood tests which can identify inherited "markers" in the blood—called "HLA antigens"—which might indicate an increased susceptibility to diabetes. This might eventually help in pinpointing women who may have an insulin problem during pregnancy.

condition called macrosomia). This is likely to mean that the baby will have to be delivered by caesarean.

After the birth the extra insulin that the baby's pancreas is producing may cause his or her blood sugar levels to fall too low (hypoglycaemia) after being separated from the rich glucose of the mother's blood. It may be necessary for the baby to be given extra glucose through an intravenous line for a while.

A woman with gestational diabetes is also more at risk of developing urinary tract infections and pre-eclampsia, a condition unique to pregnancy.

Treatment

Most pregnant women need only dietary treatment to regulate their blood glucose levels, but a few may need insulin injections. Your doctor or a dietician will help you to plan your meals—what to eat and when to eat it—to make sure that your blood glucose levels are maintained within a healthy range. Regular, gentle exercise will also help to lower your blood glucose level and prevent high blood pressure.

What causes diabetes?

Chapter

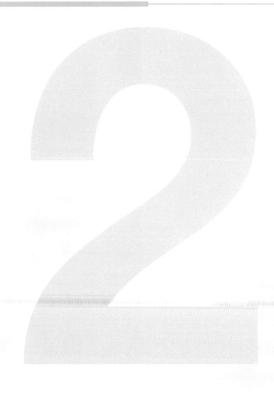

ASSESSMENT & DIAGNOSIS

Spotting the symptoms

TYPE 2: LATE-ONSET DIABETES

COMMON	POSSIBLE
◆ Feeling more thirsty than usual	◆ Genital itching
◆ More frequent urination	◆ Blurred vision
◆ Some loss of weight	
◆ Feeling tired and lacking in energy	

WARNING

Even minor symptoms may indicate raised blood glucose levels, which can cause damage over a long period of time. It is best to see your doctor, even if it turns out to be a false alarm, rather than do nothing about the symptoms you have.

TYPE 1: INSULIN-DEPENDENT DIABETES

ALWAYS	SOMETIMES
◆ Constant, severe thirst	◆ Dehydration
◆ Very frequent urination	◆ Urinary infection, cystitis
◆ Sudden and dramatic weight loss	◆ Vomiting
◆ Severe tiredness	◆ Keto-acidotic coma
◆ Blurred vision	◆ Itchy genitals

WARNING

These symptoms may become severe quite quickly, and it is important to get medical attention to prevent dehydration and the possibility of the person going into a coma.

Although people with either type of diabetes may experience some of the same symptoms, there is a difference in their severity. In addition, when the pancreas stops producing insulin altogether, as in type 1 (insulin-dependent diabetes), the individual concerned is likely go from feeling all right to feeling seriously unwell in weeks rather than months. If symptoms come on over a relatively short period in a child or young adult, consult a doctor without delay

A child or young person who develops insulin-dependent diabetes will normally be feeling very unwell and their symptoms are usually unmistakable.

Older children and teenagers can explain how they feel, but with a baby or toddler your only clues may be constant crying and weight loss.

If symptoms aren't treated...

A person with untreated type 1 diabetes can go into a keto-acidotic coma because lack of insulin causes the breakdown of body fat and muscle to provide energy, producing by-products called ketones. If this happens, he or she will probably need to be admitted to hospital to have their blood glucose brought under control and stabilized.

Since the body can't make proper use of glucose for fuel, it breaks down fat and muscle tissue to use as fuel, sometimes causing rapid and dramatic loss of weight.

In contrast, non-insulin-dependent diabetes usually develops quite slowly, often over a number of years. In this time the person affected may experience few or even no symptoms, or such mild ones that they are easily dismissed or ignored. In such cases the chance of falling into a coma are very slight.

YOU REALLY NEED TO KNOW

◆ When your body stops producing insulin you quite quickly start to feel very unwell.

◆ You may develop type 2 diabetes without having very noticeable symptoms.

◆ You are unlikely to go into a coma if you develop diabetes later in life.

Spotting the symptoms

Spotting the symptoms

✔ If any symptoms return after treatment has begun, go back to your doctor. Changes to the type of treatment or dosage may be needed.

✘ Anyone over 40 should not ignore even minor symptoms. Excessive thirst and urinating much more often need to be checked out.

It is possible for diabetes to begin causing problems in several parts of your body when you have had the condition for a number of years, especially if your blood glucose levels have not been tightly controlled.

Are complications developing?

Although regular check-ups are designed to pick up any early signs of such problems, you should report any unusual symptoms to your doctor because they may need further investigation and treatment. Those listed in the chart below, for example, may not be caused by diabetes, but if they are the sooner treatment is begun the more likely it is to be effective.

Long-term diabetes increases your risk of developing problems, such as angina, which are in any case more common in people over 50.

SYMPTOMS AND COMPLICATIONS

◆ Your eyesight changes for the worse

◆ Your feet or hands become numb or less sensitive to pain

◆ Your feet or hands seem to be permanently cold

◆ You get breathless after relatively minor exertion

◆ You have chest pains

WARNING
You should see your doctor immediately if you have any of the symptoms listed above because they may suggest that complications are developing.

SYMPTOMS AND BLOOD GLUCOSE

Regular monitoring of your blood glucose level will tell you if your treatment is not having the desired effect. If the level is consistently raised, you may find that you start to experience some of the symptoms you used to have before your condition was diagnosed, and you should consult your doctor or diabetes nurse about possible adjustments or changes.

When you are being treated with insulin and some kinds of tablets, you may have the opposite problem, experiencing different symptoms because your blood glucose regularly drops too low. Again, you should seek help from your medical advisers to sort out the problem.

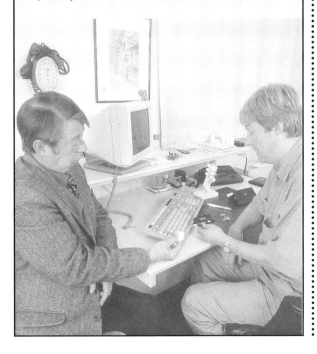

YOU REALLY NEED TO KNOW

◆ Bladder and kidney infections and thrush are more common in people who have consistently raised blood glucose levels.

◆ People with type 2 diabetes may find they have problems with their teeth and gums, and cuts and grazes heal more slowly.

Spotting the symptoms

Diagnostic tests

DOs AND DON'Ts

See your doctor if you notice any symptoms which suggest you might have diabetes.

Try not to worry if your GP suggests you have the condition as it can be controlled with the right treatment.

If you have any of the symptoms of insulin-dependent diabetes (see p. 24), your doctor will not have difficulty in diagnosing your condition. With type 2 diabetes, however, unless you have gone to your GP because you suspect you may have diabetes, your condition may be picked up by chance during a routine examination for another complaint. It is not uncommon for people who have had undiagnosed non-insulin-dependent diabetes for years to find out when an ophthalmologist notices changes in their retina during a routine sight test.

If diabetes is suspected, the GP may take blood and/or urine samples in the surgery.

Blood tests

If your GP has a blood glucose testing meter and strips he or she will be able to tell within seconds whether your glucose level is raised. Your doctor may decide that you need to have further blood tests done at hospital.

GLUCOSE IN THE URINE

A high level of urinary glucose is important and may well indicate diabetoo, but a slight rise is more difficult to assess. When your blood glucose level is above normal, some glucose may spill over into your urine, but at what point this happens varies from one person to another. This is determined by your "renal threshold".

Glucose begins to overflow into the urine because your body cannot re-absorb the amount being filtered out of your bloodstream by the kidneys. People with a low threshold may have glucose in their urine even though they do not have diabetes, but further investigations will be necessary to confirm this.

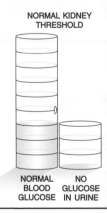

NORMAL KIDNEY THRESHOLD

NORMAL BLOOD GLUCOSE

NO GLUCOSE IN URINE

DIAGNOSING YOUNG PEOPLE

A child or young person who has clear cut symptoms of type 1 diabetes is likely to have to go into hospital straightaway. The diagnosis will be confirmed there by doctors who have particular expertise in looking after young people with the condition. Insulin treatment will probably be started immediately.

Urine tests

Doctors have simple kits to check whether there is glucose in your urine, but a sample will probably be sent to the lab for analysis anyway. As well as analysing the sample for the presence of glucose, the lab will also check for ketones, acidic compounds produced when body fat instead of carbohydrate is used as fuel.

YOU REALLY NEED TO KNOW

◆ Young people who develop type 1 diabetes will be diagnosed more quickly than an older person who has type 2.

◆ Your doctor may give you the results of blood and urine tests on the spot. You may have to wait a few days if the samples have to be sent for analysis.

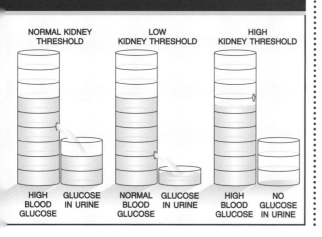

NORMAL KIDNEY THRESHOLD		LOW KIDNEY THRESHOLD		HIGH KIDNEY THRESHOLD	
HIGH BLOOD GLUCOSE	GLUCOSE IN URINE	NORMAL BLOOD GLUCOSE	GLUCOSE IN URINE	HIGH BLOOD GLUCOSE	NO GLUCOSE IN URINE

Glucose tolerance test

Whether it is done in your doctor's surgery or at the lab, measuring the level of glucose in your blood can normally confirm whether you have diabetes. However, if you have no symptoms and the level is only slightly above normal, you may have to have what's called a glucose tolerance test (GTT) before a definite diagnosis can be made. This will be done at the outpatients' clinic at your local hospital.

RESPONSE TO A GLUCOSE TOLERANCE TEST

The point of a glucose tolerance test is to distinguish between those people who are healthy despite having mildly raised blood glucose levels and those who have diabetes. The test measures your body's response to an intake of glucose over a set period of time—three hours—which gives a more accurate picture of changes in the blood.

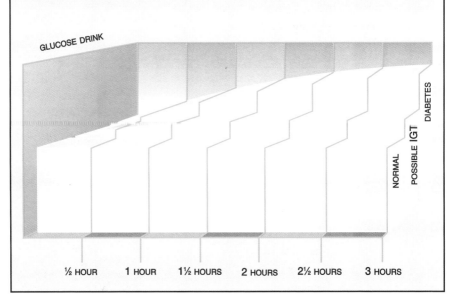

GLUCOSE DRINK

NORMAL POSSIBLE IGT DIABETES

½ HOUR   1 HOUR   1½ HOURS   2 HOURS   2½ HOURS   3 HOURS

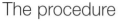

The procedure

You need to allow around three hours at the outpatients' clinic for a glucose tolerance test. You will be asked to come to the clinic first thing in the morning having had nothing to eat or drink (except water) since your meal the previous evening.

Your blood glucose will be measured and a urine sample may be taken as well, then you will be given a drink containing a known quantity of glucose.

The blood test will then be repeated every half hour over the next two hours, and you may also have to give two more urine samples, one after the first hour and one after the second.

What the results mean

The results of the blood and urine tests will show how your body has responded to the glucose which you have drunk (see illustration left). There are three possible conclusions which will clarify whether you do or don't have diabetes or have a related problem called Impaired Glucose Tolerance (IGT).

◆ 1. Your response indicates that your blood glucose levels are not above normal. You do not have diabetes.

◆ 2. Your glucose level is only slightly higher than normal, and again, this means you don't have diabetes. However, this result suggests that you have Impaired Glucose Tolerance, and can be considered at increased risk of developing diabetes in the future.

If a glucose tolerance test shows you have IGT, you will be given advice on the right kind of diet and lifestyle changes to make to prevent this happening.

◆ 3. Your glucose levels are sufficiently high to confirm the diagnosis of diabetes mellitus.

YOU REALLY NEED TO KNOW

◆ If blood and urine tests are borderline further tests may be necessary later.

◆ You should not eat or drink after your evening meal if you are having a glucose tolerance test the next morning.

Glucose tolerance test

Your medical team

✓ Talk to your diabetes specialist nurse if you need personal advice on managing your condition.

✗ The professionals can only do so much. You are best placed to monitor your health and make necessary changes to your lifestyle.

You and your family may well be shocked and upset to discover that you have diabetes, and worry about how it will affect your lives in future. It often takes time to come to terms with the diagnosis, but with the right treatment and a bit of planning, you will soon learn to manage your condition so that it interferes with everyday living as little as possible.

Who does what?

Depending on local arrangements, you may be cared for by your GP, by a team at the local hospital or by both in partnership. Many GP surgeries now run regular diabetes clinics and, especially if you have non-insulin-dependent diabetes, you may only need to go to the hospital clinic once or twice a year for thorough check-ups.

WHO'S WHO IN THE TEAM

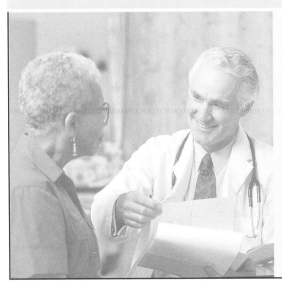

Your primary care will be in the hands of the professionals at your surgery of choice. Your GP is the first point of contact and after a diagnosis has been made the diabetes specialist nurse will give help and advice on meeting the needs of your condition and treatment. Through the surgery you can talk to a dietician about food and be referred to a podiatrist or chiropodist for feet care.

IF YOU WANT TO CHANGE YOUR GP

If you feel you would rather go to a different doctor, all you have to do is to check that the practice of your choice will accept you as a patient, and ask to be registered. They will then arrange for your records to be transferred.

After you have been diagnosed, the most important person you will see will probably be the diabetes specialist nurse, either at the surgery or the hospital. She will teach you all you need to know about doing your part in managing your condition, including monitoring your blood glucose and, if appropriate, injecting insulin. You will be able to see her as often as you need to, and she will also be available to answer any queries on the phone.

You should also be given the opportunity of a full discussion with a dietician. He or she will explain the importance of eating the right foods to control blood glucose, losing weight if necessary, and give you advice on how to adjust your daily meals.

Playing your part

However good they are, the professionals depend on you to learn as much as you can about your condition and to play a vital role in controlling it. As well as following treatment advice, you will need to monitor your blood glucose levels and make any necessary changes to your diet and lifestyle. The experts can advise you, but it's up to you to be a partner in your own care.

Controlling your diabetes requires a considerable degree of commitment, but the effort is worthwhile.

Your medical team

Chapter

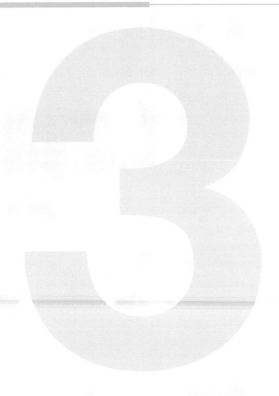

TREATMENT & CONTROL

Your diet and diabetes

✓ Carbohydrate should be the main source of energy in the diet. It is broken down by digestive enzymes into simple sugars and then enters the bloodstream.

✓ Eat plenty of fresh fruit and vegetables, and get as much of your protein from relatively low-fat sources as you can

✓ Keep sweet things to a minimum and aim to have them soon after a meal.

✗ Don't skip breakfast. It is particularly important to give your body fuel from the time you start the day.

If you have been newly diagnosed with type 2 diabetes, changing what you eat and drink may be all that is needed to keep your blood glucose under control. There are also likely to be other changes you can make to your lifestyle which will help as well. The advice will be the same whether your diabetes is treated with tablets or insulin. These are the best ways known to make your treatment successful.

The good news is that a healthy diet does not mean giving up everything you enjoy or eating different food from the rest of your family and friends. In fact, they will derive health benefits from following the same kind of eating programme as you.

You need to consider both what you eat and when you eat it. Regular meals, taken at roughly the same time each day, will help the body handle the supply of glucose and keep it in balance. It is very important not to skip meals, especially breakfast.

Cut down on fat and sugar

While there are no good or bad foods, some are certainly better for you than others. Some are high in fat that you can't see, so-called "hidden" fat which is in processed foods such as sausages, pies and burgers, bought cakes, pastries and biscuits. Ideally, you should aim to get no more than 30 percent of your daily calorie intake from fat, and most of it polyunsaturated or mono-unsaturated, rather than saturated fat. Changing over to low-fat options, such as skimmed or semi-skimmed milk, cheese and yogurt will help. Another fat-saver is grilling meat rather than frying or roasting it.

Keep sweet and sugary foods to a minimum. Choosing those made with artificial sweeteners is fine.

Enjoy carbohydrates

If you include wholemeal bread, rice, pasta and potatoes in your diet every day, you can be sure that glucose is being released comparatively slowly into your blood, which is great for controlling your condition.

Choose more fibre

Fresh vegetables, cereals, fruit and pulses such as peas and lentils will boost your fibre intake as well as providing you with important vitamins and minerals to keep you in good form. Plenty of daily fibre is essential to keep your digestive system healthy.

Pick protein carefully

If you vary the foods you eat, you will get all the protein you need. For good health, you're better off choosing poultry, eggs, fish or low-fat dairy foods rather than meat which has a high fat content. And don't forget vegetable protein; it's found in soya and other beans.

Avoid salt

Salt can aggravate any tendency to high blood pressure to which you are susceptible because you have diabetes. Never add salt when cooking or at the table, or have too many salty snacks or processed foods.

THE TYPES OF FAT

There are three categories: saturated (mostly from animal sources), un- and polyunsaturated (fish, certain vegetable oils), and mono-unsaturated (olive oil, avocados).

Healthy eating programme

DOs AND DON'Ts

✔ Include starchy carbohydrates as part of each meal and try to eat a wide variety of fresh food.

✔ Among the foods that release energy slowly are peas, beans, lentils, peaches, milk, wholegrain breads and pasta.

✗ Foods that are digested fast include bananas, raisins, carrots, potatoes, oat bran, cornflakes and white bread.

If you normally eat with your family, there is no need for this to change just because you discover that you have diabetes. They too will gain health benefits from eating the same things you do.

A well-balanced diet is one that can supply all the nutrients the body needs from adequate amounts of carbohydrate, fruit and vegetables, protein and fat. Aim to consume a wide variety of ingredients, including more

MEAL PLANNING

FOOD GROUP	INCLUDES
CARBOHYDRATES	Savoury: pasta, rice, potatoes, bread, cereals. Sweet: all kinds of sugar.
PROTEIN	All meats including poultry and game, fish, eggs and dairy foods, nuts, beans, tofu and soya.
FATS	Butter and non-butter spreads, dairy products, meats, many processed foods, cakes and pastries, cooking and salad oils.
FIBRE	All vegetables, salads and fruit, cereals, wholegrains (all of which are carbohydrate as well).

fresh foods and fewer processed ingredients and keeping fatty and sugary foods to a minimum. A diet that is high in animal fats, sugar and alcohol may raise the level of blood fats known as lipids (such as cholesterol) and can increase the risk of developing heart disease.

All foods contain calories. Some—sugar, fat and refined foods—are high in calories and have few nutrients. Those high in nutrients are best for you.

COMMENTS

Include complex (non-sugary) carbohydrates as part of every meal. They make you feel full without being fattening. Choose savoury carbohydrate-rich snacks to keep your blood glucose level balanced.

Choose low-fat dairy foods and less fatty varieties of animal protein, such as turkey and chicken. Always cook without added fat. Eat more fish. Make salads of protein vegetables, like mixed beans.

Opt for low-fat alternatives and lean cuts of meat; cut off visible fat. Eat fats sparingly. They provide little in the way of nourishment (just like sugar, salt and alcohol) and affect your blood glucose balance.

As well as potatoes or rice, aim for five portions of nutrient-rich fruit and vegetables a day. Snack on fresh fruit or raw vegetables; serve lightly cooked or grated foods in salads; combine fresh with canned fruit (in juice).

YOU REALLY NEED TO KNOW

◆ If you need to lose weight talk to a dietician about the best way of doing it.

◆ Grain foods and fruit have few calories and lots of the vitamins and minerals needed for good health.

◆ Keep foods high in refined carbohydrate and sugar for times when you need to raise your blood glucose level.

Why exercise matters

Start slowly if you are not used to exercise and get expert advice before you begin something new.

If you are susceptible to hypos, always check your blood glucose before and after any physical activity.

Even if you have never exercised before, finding out that you have diabetes may motivate you to begin once you realize how much you have to gain. Regular physical activity helps to keep your body in good working order. It tones up your muscles, increases your stamina, strength and flexibility and lifts your mood.

Heart and circulation

The kind of exercise which makes you perspire a little and leaves you breathing hard encourages your heart to pump the blood around your body and so tones up your circulation. This is especially important when you have diabetes as you are at increased risk of cardiovascular complications in the long-term.

HOW EXERCISE IMPROVES DIABETES

Muscles draw on blood glucose for fuel when you exercise and your metabolic rate rises and remains higher for some hours after. Your muscles will also need to refuel later, all of which helps to lower blood glucose levels.

AT REST

◆ Glucose and fat absorbed into the blood

◆ Insulin released from pancreas or injection site

◆ Liver stores glucose

◆ Fat stores fatty acids

◆ Muscle stores glucose.

BRIEF EXERCISE

◆ Glucose and fat absorbed into the blood

◆ Less insulin released as glucose falls

◆ Liver starts to release glucose

◆ Fat starts to release fatty acids

◆ Muscles convert stores to glucose for energy.

LONGER EXERCISE

◆ Blood diverted to muscle —less glucose and fat absorbed into the blood

◆ Less insulin released as glucose falls

◆ Liver releases a lot of glucose

◆ Fat releases lots of fatty acids

◆ Muscle takes up glucose and fatty acids for energy.

PUT SAFETY FIRST

People with diabetes can enjoy almost all types of sport and activity, but there are some points to consider:

◆ Ask the advice of your doctor or diabetes nurse before you start an exercise programme.

◆ Begin with regular moderate activity, such as walking, swimming or cycling, and only consider moving on to high-intensity activities such as squash when you are fit.

◆ Always exercise with someone else who knows what to do if you have a hypo (see p. 60).

Treatment effectiveness

Any form of treatment will work better if you exercise regularly. You may even eventually be able to reduce the dose of insulin or tablets, with your doctor's advice.

Blood glucose

Muscles will draw on glucose in your bloodstream for fuel, so the more you use them, the lower your blood glucose level is likely to be. Always check it before and after exercise, and if you are taking insulin or some forms of oral treatment, you may need to adjust the dose or take extra carbohydrate to avoid a hypo (see p. 60).

Weight loss

Exercise burns calories and increases your metabolic rate, which means that you continue to burn calories faster for some time after you have cooled down.

YOU REALLY NEED TO KNOW

◆ Exercise tailored to your abilities and level of fitness will improve your general health.

◆ Exercise may make your treatment more effective, as well as reducing the chances of some long-term complications.

◆ Carbohydrate snacks are used by athletes to maintain glucose supplies at an optimum level.

Why exercise matters

Learning to enjoy exercise

Always have some quick-acting carbohydrate easily available while exercising if you are at risk of a hypo.

Take proper precautions in any sport where you might get into difficulties, such as swimming or skiing.

If you are susceptible to hypos, take frequent blood glucose readings and be prepared to adjust your dosage and food intake.

Our bodies are designed to be exercised regularly, but modern living has made it possible for most of us to avoid physical activity entirely if we want to. Building exercise into your normal routine has undoubted health benefits, and even more so if you have diabetes.

How exercise helps you

◆ Moderate activity that leaves you slightly out of breath will tone up your heart, lungs and circulation.

◆ Your muscles use glucose as fuel, so exercise helps control the level in your bloodstream.

◆ Exercise increases your metabolic rate, so you burn calories faster. This stops you putting on the pounds and even encourages weight loss. Maintaining a weight that is right for your height will make controlling your blood glucose easier and you may even be able to reduce your medication.

Think active

You can boost your physical fitness by making small changes: try to get into new habits, such climbing stairs rather than taking the lift, and walking rather than driving to the shops.

When it comes to beginning a specific exercise programme, start slowly if you're very unfit and try to do something you actually enjoy. Dancing or yoga may be more appealing than jogging or aerobics, for example. A 20- to 30-minute brisk walk or swim three times a week would be a good start, but most forms of exercise and sports are possible provided you are sensible and don't overstrain yourself. Discuss it with your doctor.

You should aim eventually to have five 30-minute spells of exercise a week.

3

Striking a balance

It makes sense to get advice from your diabetes care team before you start any new exercise programme, but if you are on sulphonylurea tablets or insulin, you will also need to know how to adjust your treatment to avoid getting hypos during or after exercise.

In principle, you need either a lower dose than normal prior to exercise or an increased carbohydrate intake, or possibly both, depending on what you plan to do. For example, you may find you need a carbohydrate snack such as a muesli bar before and/or after exercising.

Check your blood glucose immediately before and after you exercise and again a couple of hours later and you will soon work out what adjustments you need to make to your treatment and/or food intake.

**YOU REALLY
NEED TO KNOW**

◆ Regular exercise can help you control your diabetes and reduce the risk of some long-term complications such as cardiovascular disease.

◆ While a specific programme of physical activity is especially beneficial, simply being more energetic in your everyday life yields real benefits too.

◆ Some potentially risky sports, such as scuba diving, have special rules for people with diabetes.

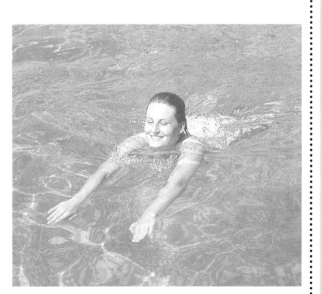

Swimming is excellent all-round exercise, using all the major muscle groups. However, diabetics should take measures to avoid a hypoglycaemic attack and never swim alone.

Learning to enjoy exercise

Oral medication

Continue taking your tablets even if you feel well.

Never stop taking tablets or change your dose without consulting your doctor.

Insulin cannot be taken by mouth as it is broken down in the digestive system. This means that in type 1 diabetes injections of insulin make up for the failure of the body's natural supply. For those people with type 2 diabetes treatment aims to help the body use the insulin that it does produce more effectively. For about 50 percent of type 2 sufferers medication in tablet form is prescribed to be used in conjunction with dietary changes.

Your doctor will usually decide on this treatment if a short period of dietary changes has not brought your blood glucose levels down into the normal range.

Oral medication for type 2 diabetes is designed to regulate blood glucose levels either by stimulating the pancreas to produce more insulin or by making that which the body produces more effective. It may take a period of experimentation to decide which kind and what

MEDICATION IN TABLET FORM

TYPE	HOW THEY WORK
SULPHONYLUREAS	Stimulate the pancreas to release more insulin
BIGUANIDES (METFORMIN)	Increases effectiveness of available insulin
ACARBOSE	Slows down digestion of starchy foods so that glucose is not released into bloodstream quickly
REPAGLINIDE (NOVONORM)	Stimulates the release of insulin in response to blood glucose levels

dosage is right for you. During this time it is important not to stop taking the tablets or change the dose without consulting your doctor or diabetes nurse.

Treatment choices

The chart below shows the four types: sulphonylureas, biguanides (metformin), alpha-glucosidase inhibitors (acarbose) and repaglinide (Novonorm). There are different formulations of sulphonylureas (SUs).

Talk to your medical team about the tablets prescribed so you know when to take them and what to expect. Find out all you can about side-effects. For example, if you are taking SUs, it is possible for your blood glucose levels to fall too low. You may be given more than one type. Acarbose, for instance, can be taken on its own or in conjunction with other oral treatments to increase their effectiveness.

POSSIBLE SIDE-EFFECTS

Low blood glucose (hypoglycaemia); flushed face after drinking alcohol; increased appetite may cause weight gain

Stomach upsets; bloating and wind in large intestine; diarrhoea

Stomach upsets

Hypos are possible but rare if tablets are always taken before meals

Oral medication

Injecting insulin

✓ If you find injections difficult or painful, ask your diabetes care team for advice.

✓ Check your injection technique with your medical advisers to make sure that the needle is going into fat rather than muscle.

✗ Don't always inject your insulin in the same place.

Everyone who has type 1 diabetes will have to have daily insulin injections for the rest of their lives. About 30 percent of people with type 2 are also treated this way. The aim of the injections is to tailor the supply of insulin as closely as possible to your individual circumstances. Your doctor or diabetes nurse will discuss with you how best to achieve this.

Self-injection

Most people find the prospect of injecting themselves a little daunting at first, but you will be given all the support you need by your medical team. Once you've mastered the technique, injecting doesn't hurt, although you may

PREPARING AN INSULIN INJECTION

◆ Attach needle to syringe if necessary.

◆ Upend the insulin bottle several times (for all except short-acting insulin).

◆ Draw air up into the syringe to the level of units you want to inject.

◆ Hold the bottle the right way up and place the needle through the top and inject air into the bottle.

◆ Hold the needle in the bottle and turn it upside down and draw the insulin into the syringe.

◆ Remove air bubbles by flicking the syringe at the bubble. When the bubble goes to the top, push the plunger to expel the air into the bottle.

WHERE TO INJECT INSULIN

There are several parts of the body where you can inject and you can choose for yourself, so long as you vary it. If you use the same spot repeatedly it may cause a fatty lump to develop which interferes with insulin absorption.

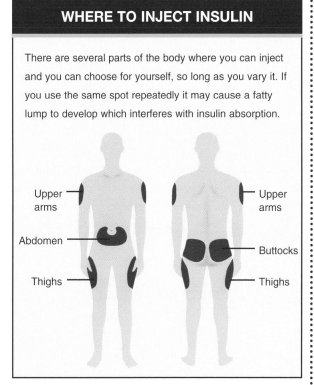

Upper arms

Abdomen

Thighs

Upper arms

Buttocks

Thighs

occasionally get a small amount of bleeding or a slight bruise if you accidentally puncture a tiny blood vessel.

A good trick to try before you inject is to first cool the skin with an ice cube. This can ease the process.

You should inject the insulin into the fatty layer under your skin, not directly into muscle. For most people, this means that the most convenient sites for injection are the abdomen and the outside of the thighs or the buttocks. Insulin injected into a fatty part of a limb may be absorbed by the body more quickly, especially if you take some exercise immediately after.

YOU REALLY NEED TO KNOW

◆ It takes takes time and practice to get used to injecting yourself.

◆ You will be helped by your doctor or diabetes nurse until you are completely confident.

◆ You and your medical advisers will decide the most appropriate schedule for you.

◆ The choices to be made include the type of insulin (how quickly it acts and how long it is effective), the number of daily injections and the delivery device.

Injecting insulin

Injecting insulin

Store insulin in the fridge between 4 and 8 °C. Bottles or cartridges in daily use will come to no harm if kept at room temperature for up to a month.

Don't leave insulin near a fire or radiator or in direct sunlight.

The types of insulin

There are three basic types of insulin used to treat diabetes: long-, medium- and short-acting. Each varies slightly in the speed at which they take effect and how long they carry on working.

Short-acting insulins are clear, the others are cloudy. So-called "mixed" insulin contains a combination of short and long-acting types, and some people who use syringes may use two different types in one injection.

"Human" insulin was introduced in 1982 and has been processed to be more or less identical to the natural form. The older types, derived from cows or pigs, are still available but people starting treatment will use human insulin.

HOW TO INJECT INSULIN

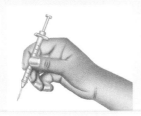

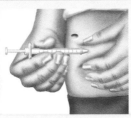

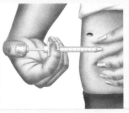

1 Hold the syringe firmly as if you were going to write with it, like a pencil.

2 With your other hand, pinch a small area of skin between your thumb and index finger. Quickly push the needle straight into the flesh at an angle of 90°, as far as it will go.

3 Still holding the flesh between finger and thumb, place your other thumb on top of the plunger and quickly and smoothly inject all the insulin from the syringe. Leave the syringe in the skin for a few seconds. Withdraw the needle straight out of the skin.

Injection regimens

When and how often you inject should be decided with your medical advisers. The best system is the one that suits you. For example, some people get on best with one daily dose of medium- or long-acting insulin, others prefer three pre-meal doses of short-acting insulin plus a bedtime one of medium-acting insulin. Still others get on better with two daily injections of combined short- and medium-acting insulin.

Injection devices

Most people who have to inject themselves use either disposable plastic syringes or an injection pen.

The pens are convenient, discreet and very easy to use: you simply load the pre-filled insulin cartridge then replace it when it's empty, or you can opt for disposable pens which are thrown away after use.

Conventional syringes come in different capacities and may be marked in steps of one or two units of insulin, so make sure you know which sort you are using. Different sizes of syringe are available, and the one you use will depend on how many units of insulin you normally take in each injection. Most syringes come with a needle attached. The needle becomes blunt after about four uses and then a new syringe is needed.

Disposing of syringes and needles

Ask your diabetes nurse about specially designed disposal units. Disposable needles used with syringes or pens can be put into a tin or plastic jar with a lid which fastens securely then thrown in the bin. Glass cartridges should be wrapped in a strong plastic or paper bag to prevent breakage before being thrown away.

YOU REALLY NEED TO KNOW

◆ The different types of insulin and injection regimens allow you to tailor your treatment to your particular lifestyle.

◆ Insulin should always be stored in a cool place.

◆ You may need to adjust your dosage as circumstances change (see p. 51).

◆ Air bubbles are not dangerous if injected, but they make the dose less accurate. If you can't remove bubbles, expel all the insulin and start again.

Injecting insulin

Monitoring blood glucose

DOs AND DON'Ts

✓ Self-monitoring of blood glucose is the only way to find out if your treatment is keeping your blood glucose within the normal range.

✗ Don't rely on guesswork or how you feel to assess your blood glucose level.

✗ Never be tempted to underestimate when reporting blood or urine test results.

It is impossible to exaggerate the importance of monitoring your blood glucose levels yourself on a regular basis. There is no other way of finding out whether your treatment is keeping your diabetes under control or whether it needs to be changed. Although you will get symptoms when your blood glucose falls too low, and may do so if it is excessively high, you cannot normally sense whether it is under control by the way you feel. Good control makes long-term complications much less likely and you will feel better when your blood glucose is within the recommended range.

If you attend the hospital outpatients' clinic for regular check-ups, you will probably have an additional blood test which analyses your blood glucose level over a longer period, but this is not an alternative to doing the recommended regular checks yourself more frequently.

Self-monitoring

There are two ways of monitoring your own blood glucose. The first, and most accurate method, involves pricking your finger to get a small drop of blood (see p. 52). The second requires testing your urine for traces of glucose which have spilled over from your bloodstream (see p. 53). If you can manage it (and most people can with some practice), testing your blood is the better option because it is more precise.

Blood glucose is measured in units called millimols per litre of blood—or mmols/l. In a person who doesn't have diabetes, the level only fluctuates between 4 and 8 mmols/l. When you have diabetes, your levels should be kept within this range for good control, but may go below or well above if not well-controlled. If this happens regularly, talk to your diabetes care team about it.

MAKING ADJUSTMENTS TO DOSAGE

If you stick to the insulin dosage recommended by your doctor and monitor your blood glucose regularly to assess its effectiveness, you will become adept at managing your diabetes. This means you will be able to make small adjustments if necessary. Remember that when you make changes, it is usually best to do so in small increments and wait two or three days to judge the effect before making further ones. You may find you need a lower dose before strenuous exercise or a higher one if you have an infection such as a cold or flu.

Accuracy is important

When your diabetes is well-controlled by diet alone, or by diet and tablets, frequent blood testing may not be essential. If, however, you are prone to hypos (see p. 60), which can happen with some kinds of tablets and with insulin, you need to have accurate information to tell you when and if your blood glucose falls too low as well as if it is too high.

The urine check may be accurate enough for some people, but others may need a different test. While it can tell you whether glucose is present, it cannot tell you how much, and if the level is too low. Your care team will advise you if a more appropriate test would be the point at which glucose spills over into the urine. This varies from one person to another, depending on your renal threshold (see p. 28).

On average, glucose overflows from the bloodstream into the urine when the level reaches 10 mmols/l.

see p. 60

see p. 28

YOU REALLY NEED TO KNOW

◆ You can monitor blood glucose either by testing your blood or by checking for the presence of glucose in your urine.

◆ Most people find measuring the glucose in blood samples accurate enough.

◆ Your diabetes care team may use the abbreviation SBGM, which simply means self blood glucose monitoring.

Monitoring blood glucose

Blood and urine tests

SELF HELP

✓ Any blood or urine test is retrospective: it records the effect of earlier meals and treatment.

✓ If your first test of the day is regularly high, consider adjusting your food intake or insulin injection the evening before.

✓ Romombor that an infection or other illness can make readings high.

Before doing a blood test wash your hands in warm water, rinsing off soap carefully. This gets rid of any residues which might affect the result and the warmth will also make the blood flow out more easily.

Prick your finger. Some people choose the fleshy area on the front and others the skin below the nailbed, but most go for the sides of the fingertips as this is least painful. Choose a different area each time you test, otherwise your fingertips can get sore.

At first you may find it difficult to draw enough blood but this usually gets better with practice. If you find the prospect of drawing blood to test off-putting, you may think it worthwhile investing in one of the special gadgets incorporating a spring-loaded lancet. You simply press a button to release the lancet and prick your finger.

HOW TO TEST YOUR BLOOD

There are several different methods for measuring your blood glucose levels, including various digital meters which provide accurate readouts. Most rely on the deposit of a blood droplet on to a test strip or pad. The most basic (and cheapest) method is to use special test strips which give a colour reading.

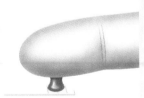

1 Deposit a small drop of blood on a testing strip so that it covers both test pads. Do not touch the strip with your finger.

TESTING YOUR URINE

This is done with testing strips which are similar to those used for blood testing. The time it takes for any colour change to develop varies with the type of strip, so check the instructions carefully.

◆ The urine you pass first thing is not a reliable indicator.

◆ You should test a sample half an hour or so after you have emptied your bladder for the first time that day.

◆ Dip a testing strip into a sample of fresh urine.

◆ Check any colour change against the chart provided.

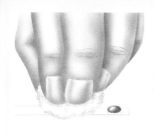
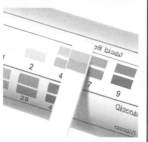
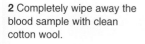

2 Completely wipe away the blood sample with clean cotton wool.

3 Compare the colour of the sample, which changes according to the glucose content, with a special chart and record the result.

YOU REALLY NEED TO KNOW

◆ Urine testing can be used to monitor blood glucose levels, but blood testing is more accurate.

◆ Occasional high or low readings are not significant, but get advice if they are consistently out of line.

◆ Spring-loaded lancet devices and electronic measuring meters may be a good investment for people who need to do regular blood glucose tests.

Blood and urine tests

Hospital check-ups

DOs AND DON'Ts

✓ Always keep your check-up appointments, even if home testing tells you your diabetes is well-controlled.

✗ Do not treat hospital tests as an alternative to self-testing.

Most people with diabetes will need to attend a hospital outpatients' clinic at least once a year for a thorough check-up and assessment. One type of test which will be conducted is designed to measure your average blood glucose level over the weeks before your visit.

Why they are done

Hospital tests complement the ones you do yourself to monitor fluctuations in blood glucose over relatively short periods. Even if you have noticed a few unusually high or unusually low readings in your home tests, the long-term assessment will reveal whether and how well your treatment is working as a whole.

While they cannot be used to make daily adjustments, these tests are useful in helping your medical advisers to decide whether any change in treatment is needed. For example, a high reading on one of these tests in a person who has been following a healthy eating programme meticulously might be a sign that they now need extra help, in the form of tablets, to keep their blood glucose under good control.

There are two tests—haemoglobin A_1 and fructosamine—both of which can also be done at other times if your doctor feels that the additional information they provide may be helpful in assessing or adjusting your treatment.

Haemoglobin A_1

The chemical haemoglobin which carries oxygen in the blood also gives red cells their colour. The tests, referred to by the abbreviation HbA_1 or HbA_1c, depending on the version being done, check whether haemoglobin and glucose have become chemically combined.

Many diabetes clinics today use the more refined version called HbA_1c, but the purpose is the same. The red blood cells which carry haemoglobin and combine with glucose have a life span of two to three months. The test indicates to your medical team what your average blood glucose levels were over that period and give an overall picture of how well your diabetes has been controlled. You will be able to discuss with them what this may mean in managing your condition.

Fructosamine

An analysis of certain proteins in the blood plasma which bind with glucose is done to provide an average of your blood glucose levels over the preceding two to three weeks. This test may be done more frequently in pregnancy to ensure that adjustments to the woman's insulin regimen are working well.

WHAT DOES IT MEAN?

WORD	MEANING
HAEMOGLOBIN	The pigment in the blood which carries oxygen and gives blood its red colour.
BLOOD PLASMA	The straw-coloured fluid which transports all the various components of the blood, such as red and white corpuscles (cells) and platelets.

YOU REALLY NEED TO KNOW

◆ Special blood tests which assess the effectiveness of your treatment over previous weeks are a normal part of your hospital check-up.

◆ The tests can be useful at other times, such as when there is a possibility your treatment may need changing.

Chapter

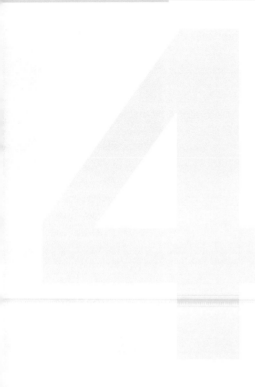

LIVING WITH DIABETES

Understanding hypoglycaemia

Try to pinpoint the
cause of hypos so
you can prevent them
happening again.

Remember that
alcohol and exercise
can make your
blood glucose levels
fall over the next
few hours.

Try not to worry about
the occasional hypo. It
is bound to happen if
your blood glucose is
tightly controlled.

If your diabetes is treated with either sulphonylurea
tablets or insulin, there is the possibility that your blood
glucose could fall too low causing a hypoglycaemic
reaction, or hypo as it is known. No matter how careful
you are about managing your condition, you will
probably experience a hypo at some time.

Symptoms of a hypo

The symptoms experienced are the result of the body
shifting essential glucose to the vital and sensitive
organs which need it, the brain in particular. The
combination of symptoms and their severity varies from
one person to another.

A few people don't get any warning signs at all. Many
find their symptoms are fairly consistent, allowing them
to recognize the onset of a hypo. Some people find that
their symptoms change or disappear altogether after
they have had diabetes for a number of years.

◆ Sweating
◆ Feeling cold and clammy
◆ Blurred vision
◆ Shakiness and trembling
◆ Tingling lips
◆ Feeling very hungry
◆ Feeling angry or irritable
◆ Pallor
◆ Vagueness or confusion
◆ Inability to concentrate
◆ If your blood glucose continues to fall,
   you may lose consciousness.

People who do not know about diabetes may mistake
some of the symptoms of a hypo for drunkenness so
don't hesitate to explain what is wrong to strangers.

When and why

A hypo occurs when you have too much insulin in your bloodstream in relation to the amount of glucose. The only solution is to correct this imbalance.

If you are having frequent hypos, you should go back to your diabetes care team and discuss why they are happening. You may need some adjustment to your treatment in order to sort the problem out. If, however, they only happen occasionally it is usually possible to identify the reason yourself with a bit of thought.

Research has shown that people who manage to achieve tight control over their blood glucose are more likely to experience the occasional hypo than those whose condition is poorly controlled.

People whose diabetes is treated with diet alone or with oral metformin or acarbose are not at risk of experiencing hypos. People taking Novonorm are unlikely to have them if they take their tablets correctly.

WHAT WENT WRONG?

Usually a hypo will be as a result of one or more of the following circumstances:

◆ Postponing or missing a meal.

◆ Taking too much insulin.

◆ A sudden burst of exercise—such as running to catch a train or bus.

◆ Drinking a lot of alcohol—especially if you did not eat some carbohydrate at the same time.

YOU REALLY NEED TO KNOW

◆ People treated with sulphonylurea tablets or insulin are at risk of hypoglycaemic attacks when their blood glucose falls below a certain level.

◆ Frequent or unexplained hypos may mean your treatment needs to be adjusted.

Preventing a hypo

✓ Always carry some form of fast-acting carbohydrate such as dextrose tablets to take as soon as you have any symptoms.

✓ Make sure that colleagues and friends know what to do if you are unable to help yourself during a hypo.

✗ Do not be afraid to ask for help if you need it. People may misunderstand your condition and not know what to do.

Although a hypo can be a very unpleasant experience and may be alarming, it does not do any actual damage to your body. Even if you lose consciousness, your body will eventually release glucose stored in the liver and raise the level in your bloodstream.

However, letting nature take its course in this way will leave you feeling unwell, as if you have a bad hangover. It is best to intervene to prevent a severe reaction.

Helping yourself

Once you notice your warning signs, take action quickly to prevent the hypo. This means drinking or eating some quick-acting sugary carbohydrate. It can be a can of sweet fizzy drink, fruit juice, a chocolate bar, a few sweets or glucose tablets. (Bear in mind that "diet" or "light" fizzy drinks contain no sugar so will not reverse the symptoms of a hypo.) This will give your blood glucose a short-term boost and should be followed with a starchy snack or a meal—for example, a sandwich, beans on toast, fresh fruit, biscuits and milk or a bowl of cereal—to stabilize the blood glucose levels and prevent another dip.

NIGHT TIME HYPOS

If you regularly wake in the morning feeling starving hungry or with hangover symptoms, you may be having night-time hypos. You can find out if this is so by doing a blood test around 3 am and then discuss adjusting your treatment with your medical advisers. A long-acting carbohydrate snack (eg, toasted cheese on rye bread) before you go to bed will help to prevent a night hypo.

EMERGENCY INJECTION

A severe hypo resulting in unconsciousness can be treated with an injection of a hormone, glucagon, which raises blood glucose levels but it needs to be given by someone trained by the diabetes care team.

What others can do

Most of the time you will recognize what is happening and be able to take the appropriate action, but occasionally you may need help from someone else.

It is useful to know that becoming irritable and awkward can be a symptom of a hypo just as much as sweating or blurred vision. This may cause you to become annoyed with anyone who suggests you should eat something or refuse to acknowledge that you're having a hypo! It's in your own interests to explain this to people with whom you spend a lot of time, such as work or team mates, so they are not put off trying to help you if you need it.

If the reaction happens very fast or without the normal warning signs, you may lose consciousness or even have a convulsion, although both are relatively rare.

Unless those around you realize what has happened, you may well wake up in an ambulance or in the Accident and Emergency department of your local hospital.

Some diabetics carry a special sugar-based gel which will reverse a hypo if smeared on to the gums. The British Diabetic Association recommends that, unless the person can still swallow, this should only be given to an unconscious person by a trained health professional.

◆ Often there are easily recognizable warning signs that a hypo is happening.

◆ Occasionally a hypo can happen very quickly and lead to loss of consciousness.

◆ A hypo has no permanent after effects, but it is unpleasant and should be nipped in the bud whenever possible.

Preventing a hypo

What about hyperglycaemia?

✓ Ask your diabetes care team what to do in the event of illness before it happens.

✓ If your blood glucose readings remain high, seek medical advice.

✗ If your diabetes is treated with insulin do not stop having your injections even if you are not eating normally.

✗ Occasional high blood glucose readings are not a cause for concern, but should be noted.

If you are doing regular blood or urine tests as you should be, you will know when your glucose levels are too high. Everyone gets the odd high reading from time to time, but if the levels are consistently above normal you need to do something about it. High blood glucose, or hyperglycaemia, means that even though you may feel quite well your diabetes is not properly controlled and action is needed to correct the situation.

For some people whose condition may be well controlled most of the time, there are some situations where their blood glucose readings may suddenly rise:

◆ It is a common response to illness, especially infections such as a cold or flu, and stomach upsets which make you feel nauseous or vomit.

◆ Some women find that their blood glucose tends to rise at certain points in their menstrual cycle or when they start taking oral contraceptives.

◆ Some people find that their blood glucose levels rise in very hot weather.

When you're not well

Any infection can cause a rise in blood glucose, because this is part of the body's defence mechanism. It can happen too if you are not eating well.

Check your blood glucose levels frequently (about four times a day), even if you don't much feel like it. If you are not well enough to do your tests, ask someone else to do them for you and to write down the results.

If you are on insulin, you may need to increase the number of units you inject each time to combat raised blood sugar levels. Your tests will tell you if this is necessary, but if you are not confident about adjusting your dose, get advice from your doctor or diabetes nurse.

Though you may not feel like eating or are being sick, keep up your carbohydrate intake with sweet milky or fizzy drinks. You should continue to have the usual number of injections even if you miss meals.

If you are vomiting

If you have any illness which makes it impossible for you to keep even fluids down contact your doctor straightaway. It is more difficult to adjust the dose of tablets yourself when you're ill, and if you are unable to eat or drink normally you should get medical advice.

Hospital treatment

Occasionally, people with type 2 diabetes may need to go into hospital in order to be treated with insulin for a few days if some other illness disrupts their normal control routine.

Help children quickly

The very young often become ill more quickly than adults, so don't delay getting advice from your GP. Regular testing is particularly important for children when they are ill.

SYMPTOMS ARE GRADUAL

Your blood glucose levels normally have to rise well above normal before you experience any symptoms. The process is gradual, so if you test your blood or urine regularly you should be able to identify the problem and take action before you start to feel any ill effects.

YOU REALLY NEED TO KNOW

◆ Respiratory and other infections can raise blood glucose levels and you may need to adjust your treatment.

◆ People with diabetes can have an annual flu jab because of the risk that such an infection will disrupt their blood glucose control.

What about hyperglycaemia?

Possible complications

✓ It is essential to have regular eye checks by a suitably qualified practitioner to ensure that any early signs of damage can be found and treated as early as possible.

✓ Take precautions to avoid accidental damage to your feet and check them daily for signs of injury or infection.

✗ Never prick a blister because this may cause an infection to enter the broken skin.

It is unfortunately the case that you may develop other conditions linked to your diabetes, although this is less likely if it has been well controlled. However, even when this does happen, there is much that can be done by way of treatment.

Feet facts

People who have had undiagnosed non-insulin-dependent diabetes for many years and those whose blood glucose has been poorly controlled are particularly prone to problems with their feet.

You need to take special care of your feet as they are vulnerable to damage of either the blood supply (narrowed arteries/atherosclerosis) or to the sensory nerves (neuropathy). A poor blood supply means your feet respond less well to extremes of temperature or to any injury or infection. When there is nerve damage, you may not notice small injuries and as a result infection can set in if you don't make a point of checking your feet for even trivial damage every day.

Anyone who has trouble with corns or bunions should see a state registered podiatrist, or chiropodist as they used to be called. He or she can also give general advice on the right way to care for your feet. Do not treat them yourself with corn plasters because these contain an acid which may increase the risk of infection.

Watch for infections

You need to take special care to avoid infections in your feet, particularly if you have reduced sensation which may prevent you noticing that infection has set in. Ultimately, a severe untreated infection could lead to gangrene. Damage to the blood supply in the feet,

FOOTCARE CHECKLIST

◆ Never neglect injuries to your feet, no matter how slight.

◆ Check your feet daily and consult a podiatrist or chiropodist about any problems. If it is difficult for you to check your own feet, get someone else to help.

◆ Wash your feet every day with soap and warm water. Do not use hot water.

◆ Dry your feet thoroughly, paying particular attention to the area between the toes.

◆ If your skin is dry or rough apply a moisturizing cream such as E45.

◆ Change your socks, tights or stockings daily.

◆ Do not wear ill-fitting shoes.

◆ Check that there is nothing in your shoes that will rub.

◆ Wear new shoes for a short time at first and check your feet afterward for any signs of rubbing.

◆ Cut your toenails following the shape of the end of your toes. Do not cut deep into the corners.

◆ Avoid extremes of temperature (for example, do not put your feet on a hot water bottle to warm them).

especially in older people with hardening or clogging of the arteries, also increases the risk of gangrene. Always go and see your doctor or diabetes nurse if an infection does not clear up on its own in a few days.

YOU REALLY NEED TO KNOW

◆ Untreated or poorly controlled diabetes can lead to problems with your eyes and feet.

◆ People with diabetes are particularly at risk of cataracts and retina damage.

◆ Consultations with a podiatrist are free to anyone with diabetes and are essential if poor eyesight or overweight makes it difficult to care for your feet.

Possible complications

Possible complications

Retinopathy

This problem can result from damage to blood vessels at the back of the eye which serve the retina. Small blisters may form in the vessel wall then burst, causing bleeding, or the blood vessels themselves may become leaky. If nothing is done, new and fragile blood vessels may grow in an attempt to restore a normal blood supply to the retina and they too may bleed.

The good news is that if these changes are picked up at an early stage, they can be treated effectively with lasers. Such treatment stops further damage occurring and usually prevents your sight getting any worse. This is why it is important for people with diabetes to have regular eye checks at least once a year. They are normally done at the hospital outpatients' clinic.

Cataracts

The lens of the eye may gradually become opaque so preventing you from seeing clearly. It is mainly due to changes that come with age, but people with diabetes are more susceptible or may develop cataracts at a younger age. Surgery to insert a replacement lens is simple and effective and can often be done without you needing to stay in hospital.

Heart disease

There is a wide range of drugs available to treat heart disease, and new ones are being introduced all the time. Depending on the exact nature of your problem, you may need to take more than one type.

Blocked arteries can often be opened up by a surgical procedure called angioplasty, while bypass operations can replace arteries that are damaged beyond repair. Even after an actual heart attack, many people make a good recovery and are able to return to normal living.

Kidney disease

When a protein called albumin is detected in your urine, it may be a sign of kidney disease caused by diabetes. As well as taking steps to ensure that your treatment keeps your blood glucose levels within the normal range, you may also be prescribed tablets designed to lower blood pressure. This is partly because high blood pressure is often associated with kidney problems, but also because such treatment may prevent or slow further damage. If the disease becomes severe enough to stop the kidneys working, the task of cleaning the blood can be taken over by a dialysis machine or it may be possible to have a kidney transplant.

High blood pressure

It is particularly important that your blood pressure is measured regularly. If it is raised, you will be given advice on changing your diet and lifestyle to try to bring it down. You may also need drug treatment, and it is important to take this as prescribed, even though you have no actual symptoms, otherwise you are at risk of a stroke.

Impotence

Damage to the blood vessels and/or the nerves supplying the penis may cause impotence in men who have had diabetes for many years especially if it has not been well controlled. Though you may feel embarrassed to discuss it with your doctor, he or she can offer a number of possible treatments, including Viagra.

YOU REALLY NEED TO KNOW

◆ The purpose of regular check-ups is to prevent complications developing.

◆ If there are early signs of complications, making extra effort to keep tight control of your blood glucose levels may prevent them from getting any worse.

◆ Taking certain supplements (such as fish oil or an appetite suppressor) can affect glucose levels. Check with the pharmacist.

Possible complications

Avoiding complications

Enlist the support of your diabetes care team as well as your nearest and dearest to help you change to a healthier lifestyle.

Try to accept your diabetes as something you have to take account of without letting it rule your life.

Don't be tempted to ignore early signs of complications hoping they will go away. Prompt treatment is essential to stop problems worsening.

Untreated or poorly controlled diabetes can lead to a variety of conditions affecting different body systems. Maintaining tight control of your blood glucose levels is the best preventative measure. A healthy eating plan and regular exercise should help to minimize your chances of developing heart and blood vessel disease. This becomes more important as you get older when damage to the cardiovascular system is likely to reveal itself with problems such as angina, heart attacks and stroke.

There are other lifestyle changes that you can make too which, while they are not guaranteed to prevent complications, can shift the odds in your favour.

Stop smoking

Even if you already have some damage, you will still benefit from stopping. All the possible complications of diabetes are more likely to affect people who smoke.

ACTION PLAN

There are plenty of things that you can do for yourself to help reduce the likelihood of complications developing.

◆ Keep tight control on your blood glucose levels.

◆ Stop smoking.

◆ Drink alcohol only in moderation.

◆ Take regular exercise.

◆ Follow a healthy, balanced diet.

◆ Watch your weight.

BE PREPARED

Keep everything involved in your treatment in one place, in a box or cupboard, and always out of reach of children. Always carry with you what you need for the day and for emergencies (glucose, diabetic card, doctor's number).

Smoking makes you more susceptible to the eye and kidney problems linked with diabetes. Cigarette smoke also increases the risk of all kinds of cardiovascular disease, cancer and other illnesses. If you feel you can't manage alone, consult your doctor about nicotine patches and other aids to giving up.

Alcohol in moderation

You can have a glass or two of wine or a pint of beer when you feel like it, but don't overdo it. Do not drink on an empty stomach. At the very least try to have some carbohydrate nibbles at the same time. Remember that alcohol can lower your blood glucose, putting you at risk of a hypo if you're on insulin or sulphonylurea tablets.

Diet

The food you eat makes an important contribution to keeping your diabetes under control. Eating little and often during a day will prevent blood glucose levels dropping dangerously. Choosing the foods that convert slowly to energy is best (see What is the glycaemic index? p. 71). If you find the adjustment difficult, try taking one step at a time, cutting down on high-fat foods and gradually adding in more fresh fruit and vegetables.

YOU REALLY NEED TO KNOW

◆ Lifestyle changes can help to prevent complications from developing.

◆ Smoking carries even bigger health risks when you have diabetes, adding to your susceptibility to heart and blood vessel disease.

◆ See your doctor if you have symptoms such as chest pain and breathlessness after even slight physical effort.

Avoiding complications

Alternative therapy

Always check that a complementary practitioner belongs to a reputable organization and has completed a recognized form of training.

Never accept treatment from anyone who promises you a cure for your diabetes or suggests you stop taking your prescribed treatment.

Many people who have a condition which cannot yet be cured by orthodox medicine are tempted to believe that one or more types of complementary therapies may hold more promise. The fact is that none of them have been shown to affect diabetes, either in the short- or long-term, and certainly you should never use any of them in preference to the treatment prescribed by your doctor.

Many pharmaceutical drugs—including metformin—were originally synthesized from plants, and researchers are currently testing a range of traditional herbal remedies said to be beneficial for people with type 2 diabetes. However, none has yet produced an effective treatment, and you should remember that treating yourself with untested herbal remedies could be potentially dangerous. Consult a qualified medical herbalist to find out what this treatment has to offer.

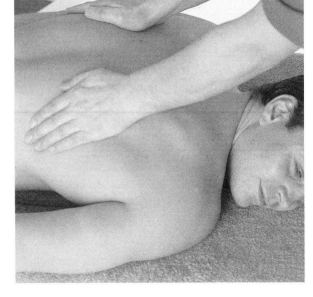

Massage with aromatherapy oils, in which the essential oils are mixed with a base or carrier oil, is an enjoyable way to relax. Applied directly to the skin in this way, the oils can have a powerful relaxing effect and help relieve stress.

WHAT IS THE GLYCAEMIC INDEX?

Some alternative therapists suggest that people with diabetes can benefit from planning their diet by taking account of the glycaemic index (GI) of individual foods.

The GI is the rate at which a food is converted into glucose in the bloodstream and the theory is that, by choosing those with a low GI, you should be able to avoid sudden rises in blood glucose. The principle lies behind the advice to include starchy savoury foods (complex carbohydrate) in every meal: wholegrains, beans, pulses, fruit and vegetables, plus meat and fish. Avoiding large amounts of sugary foods (refined carbohydrate) is also important, such as any containing maltose, glucose, corn syrup, lactose, sucrose. To apply the GI in practice can time time and effort—and is easier if you prepare all your meals at home along healthy eating guidelines (see p. 36).

Helping mind and body

While complementary therapies cannot increase your insulin supply or improve your response to it, some people find that treatments such as massage, aromatherapy and reflexology or techniques such as yoga and meditation can make it easier to live with their diabetes. You may find that different forms of therapy which relieve psychological stress or help you to cope better with your condition are worth trying, so long as you can afford it and don't expect miracles. You should be able to find classes, such as yoga, meditation and relaxation, locally. There is also a wide range of books, tapes and videos you can buy to use at home.

**YOU REALLY
NEED TO KNOW**

◆ There is no complementary therapy which can restore a failed or diminishing insulin supply or affect insulin resistance.

◆ Herbal and other remedies have not been tested for effectiveness or safety in the same way as conventional drugs.

◆ Complementary therapy which improves your sense of wellbeing or reduces stress can be beneficial provided you are realistic about what to expect from it.

Alternative therapy

Special situations

Diabetes is a serious medical condition but it should not restrict your lifestyle severely. You will be able to cope with most things with a little advance planning.

Pregnancy and birth

Most women with diabetes have problem-free pregnancies and normal healthy babies, provided their blood glucose levels are well-controlled. All will take insulin by injection while pregnant.

Even if your blood glucose control has not been perfect prior to conception, you will be strongly advised to do more monitoring and adjust your insulin doses as necessary to ensure your levels remain under control throughout your pregnancy and don't adversely affect the baby's weight. This usually requires considerably more insulin than you usually take.

You may be able to have a normal labour, though it may be necessary to give you insulin and glucose through drips to keep your blood glucose balanced. If the level is too high, your baby will produce extra insulin to cope and may be born with hypoglycaemia, but this will quickly resolve itself.

Travelling abroad

The fact that you have diabetes need not affect your travel plans in any way provided you take a few commonsense precautions.

If you are travelling by air, carry all your medication and monitoring equipment in your hand luggage and keep it with you. Don't run the risk of insulin freezing in the aircraft hold, or baggage going astray. When you're staying in a hot climate, store your spare insulin in a fridge if you can, or otherwise keep it as cool as possible.

You may like to consult your doctor or diabetes nurse about whether you will need to adjust your treatment doses while you're away, especially if you are flying a long distance. This won't usually be necessary for people on tablets but those on insulin may have to adjust their injection regimen to take account of time changes.

Many people find that their blood glucose levels change on holiday—especially in hot weather or when they are walking or swimming most days, for example. Tummy upsets can be a particular nuisance when you have diabetes, so do be extra careful about what and where you eat and drink.

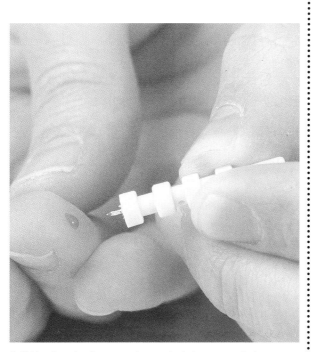

Self blood testing becomes increasingly important during pregnancy, with more frequent monitoring so that the baby grows well and healthily without undue weight gain.

◆ Raised blood glucose during pregnancy causes the baby to gain too much weight and may mean a premature delivery.

◆ Although many airlines provide so-called "diabetic" meals if you ask in good time, you will normally be able to eat the ordinary meals provided.

◆ When travelling long distances keep yourself well hydrated with plain water and avoid drinking alcohol.

Special situations

Who you should tell

✓ Make sure that any health professional treating you for another condition knows that you have diabetes.

✓ Tell the DVLA and your vehicle insurance company that you have diabetes and if you change to a different type of treatment.

✓ Tell colleagues and people you exercise or play sport with, especially if you are susceptible to hypos.

✓ Before taking out a travel insurance policy, check that it doesn't exclude "pre-existing" conditions or problems resulting from your diabetes won't be covered.

You may not want everyone to know that you have diabetes, but there are certain situations where it is in your own interests to tell people, and a few where you are actually required to do so.

Medical and dental treatment

Your GP will have details of your diabetes on your medical records, but it makes sense to remind him or her when you are being seen because of some unrelated symptoms or condition, especially if you are not seeing your usual doctor. You should also remind any doctor who treats you in hospital, especially if you are in Accident and Emergency department and they have no notes about you.

Your dentist will probably ask before beginning treatment, but if not, mention your diabetes yourself.

When your treatment changes

Both sulphonylurea tablets and insulin mean that you may have a hypo at some point, so when you start taking either for the first time, it is important that those people with whom you spend a lot of time know the signs and what action to take if necessary.

You should also tell team mates if you play sport, the teacher at any kind of exercise class and anyone who's with you in a situation where you might have an unexpected hypo.

Similarly if you get warning signs of a hypo, tell someone in case you suddenly need help to counteract low blood glucose. Always carry glucose tablets as well as quick carbohydrate snacks such as a muesli bar, and make sure they are easily accessible. Tell others where they are and when and why you may need them.

At work

Your employer and colleagues may need to know as there may be restrictions relating to potentially dangerous environments and some jobs may no longer be open to you. In any case, colleagues may need to understand why it is important for you to eat at regular times, limit your drinking and so on.

What other people need to know

Colleagues and friends may need to know about your diabetes if you are being treated with insulin or tablets which make you susceptible to hypos. Explain what they are, describing the possible symptoms, and what others should do to help. Tell them where you keep your glucose tablets or to get you a sweet drink should the need arise. You might need to explain that it is important for you to eat proper meals at particular times, so lunchtime meetings or working late may be difficult for you.

IF YOU ARE A DRIVER

YOU MUST TELL THE DVLA

As this is the authority which issues your driving licence you will be asked to provide medical information including whether you are on insulin. Your licence will not be issued for life but for a period of up to three years at a time. Restrictions may be imposed on the type of vehicles you can drive.

YOU MUST TELL YOUR VEHICLE INSURERS:

It may not affect your cover or premium, but failure to supply medical information may make your cover invalid.

◆ Some people and organizations need to know that you suffer from diabetes.

◆ You can contact the BDA for advice if you feel your employers are discriminating against you unfairly because of your condition.

◆ The easiest way to protect yourself in an emergency is to carry an identity card (available from the BDA, see p. 78) or wear a special bracelet or necklace with details of your condition.

Who you should tell

Understanding the jargon

When your diabetes is first diagnosed, you are likely to have to learn a whole new vocabulary so that you will understand what your medical advisers are telling you. It will take time to absorb all the new information, but you'll be surprised at how quickly you start to use these terms and how they no longer seem strange.

ACARBOSE—a tablet treatment for type 1 diabetes which slows the digestion of carbohydrates.

ALBUMIN—a protein sometimes found in urine, whose presence may indicate kidney damage.

ANGINA—pain in the chest and possibly the arms caused by a restricted blood supply to the heart resulting from narrowed arteries.

FRUCTOSAMINE—a blood test performed in hospital which measures average blood glucose levels over the preceding two to three weeks.

HBA$_1$(C)—a hospital blood test which measures the average blood glucose levels over the preceding two to three months.

HYPERGLYCAEMIA—above normal blood glucose levels.

HYPOGLYCAEMIA—low levels of blood glucose which trigger unpleasant symptoms and may cause loss of consciousness if not corrected.

KETONES—breakdown products found in the urine as a result of excessively high blood glucose levels. They smell of acetone or pear drops and make the blood acid.

METFORMIN—tablet treatment for type 2 diabetes which alters glucose absorption by helping insulin to work rather than affecting insulin production.

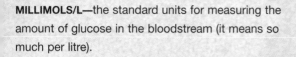

MILLIMOLS/L—the standard units for measuring the amount of glucose in the bloodstream (it means so much per litre).

NEUROPATHY—damage to the nerves, especially in the legs and feet, which may be a long-term complication of diabetes.

NOVONORM—repaglinide tablets for type 2 diabetes which stimulate insulin production.

PANCREAS—a small gland near the stomach and the liver which secretes insulin as well as other hormones and digestive enzymes.

RENAL THRESHOLD—the point at which excess blood glucose spills into the urine because it cannot be reabsorbed by the kidneys.

RETINOPATHY—damage to the blood vessels supplying the retina at the back of the eye.

SBGM—self blood glucose monitoring.

STARCHES—the most important carbohydrate for healthy eating. They take longer to be broken down by the digestive processes and to be absorbed into the bloodstream as glucose.

SULPHONYLUREAS—tablet treatments for type 2 diabetes which stimulate the release of insulin, thus lowering blood glucose.

Understanding the jargon

Useful addresses

WHERE TO GO FOR HELP

Your doctors and diabetes specialist nurses are the ones who know you and your condition best and can give you specific advice about how best to manage your condition.

BRITISH DIABETIC ASSOCIATION
10 Queen Anne Street
London W1M 0BD
Web site: http://www.diabetes.org.uk
email: careline@diabetes.org.uk

Everyone with diabetes can get valuable additional information and advice by becoming a member of the British Diabetic Association, the leading charity which is changing its name to Diabetes UK. As well as a wide range of publications on every aspect of the condition, they publish Balance magazine for members six times a year and offer a range of financial services for members.
You can also get general health advice by calling the BDA Careline: 020 7636 6112 (9–5 Mon-Fri).
You can also write to Careline at the address above.

MEDICALERT FOUNDATION,
1 Bridge Wharf,
156 Caledonian Road,
London N1 9UU.
FREEPHONE: 0800 581420

MedicAlert is a charity which sells bracelets and necklaces inscribed with important information about your diabetes and treatment which may be vital if you are ill or injured and unable to give this information yourself. Write or phone for details of membership and products.

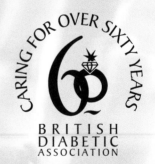

Index

Index

Acknowledgements

Photographs: BSIP Barrelle/SPL, p. 43; BSIP Krassovsky/Science Photo Library (SPL), pp. 8–9, 19;
Tony Craddock/SPL, pp. 38–39; Simon Fraser/SPL, p. 27; Jerrican Laguet/SPL, pp. 34–35, 41;
Damien Lovegrove/SPL, p. 65; Robert Harding Picture Library, pp. 22-23; Saturn Stills/SPL, pp. 53, 63, 73;
Telegraph Colour Library, pp32; Jerome Yeats/SPL, pp. 56–57
Illustrations: Kuo Kang Chen, pp. 13, 14, 17, 47, 48, 52–53; Martin Laurie, pp. 10, 28–29, 30, 40.